Self-Massage:

How to Relieve Stress with Self-Massaging Techniques

Disclaimer

Table of Contents

Introduction

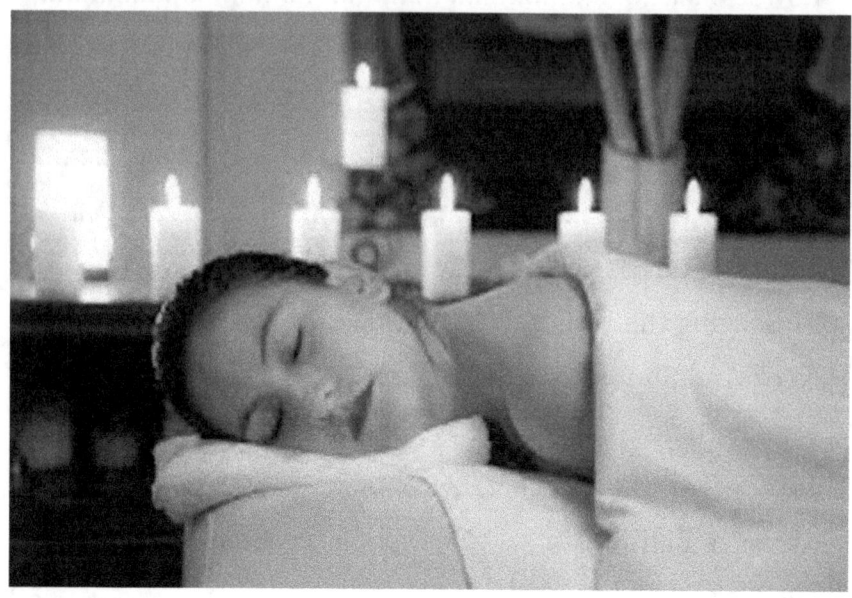

Indulging in a massage is perhaps one of the oldest ways of relieving the body's aches and stresses. Unfortunately, finding a good masseuse isn't always a luxury that everyone can afford. And that's where self-massage comes in. Consider self-massage as the epitome of self-care after a long, tired day of work. With the right tools and techniques, massage therapy should soothe your sore muscles in no time. Depending on your skill level, a session of self-massage can relax aching muscles, relieve headaches and counter stress. All of which will inevitably contribute to better well-being. So, what are you waiting for? Let's get started!

Benefits of Self Massage

Giving yourself a relaxing massage isn't as complicated as you might think. In fact, it is a habit that should become second nature, if you want to lead a healthy life. Some of the benefits of self-massage include:

Increased Blood Circulation
A gentle massage increases blood circulation, which contributes to better health. Additionally, self-massage can be beneficial for toning muscles and calming your nerves.

Therapeutic Benefits
Aside from the many physical benefits of indulging in a massage, a couple of minutes of self-care can produce feelings of relaxation, all the lotions and potions needed offering a range of therapeutic benefits.
However, it should be noted that self-massaging does not serve as a replacement for proper medical care. Make sure you speak to a professional if you are suffering from health problems.

Increased Mental Alertness
After a few sessions, you are likely to experience increased mental alertness and clarity. Self-massaging can also boost levels of stamina and curb insomnia, contributing to better mental health.

How to Create a Soothing Environment

While there are many proven health benefits of giving yourself a relaxing massage, it's best to start by creating your own little sanctuary. It is essential you choose a space that is clean, well-stocked with necessary equipment and has a relaxing environment.

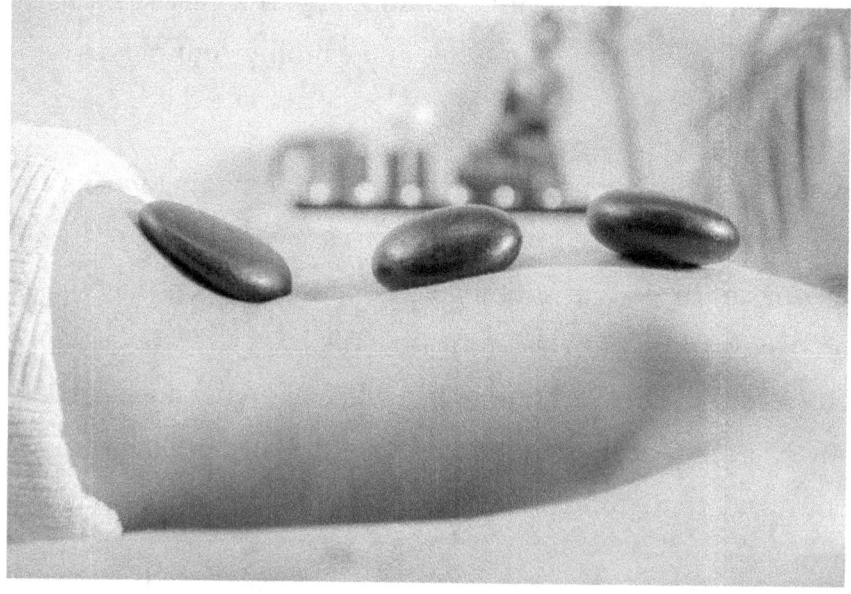

Make sure to switch off your phone and get rid of any kind of unwanted distractions that might ruin the good vibes.

Here are some simple ways to create a relaxing ambiance at home:

Lighting

Factors such as lighting may seem unimportant, but it really can play an important role in setting the right ambience. Harsh lighting can be a cause of irritation, so why not set the mood with low-lit lamps and lights. Another tip is to keep the colors and shades of the room in mind while considering which lighting to choose.

Calming Scents

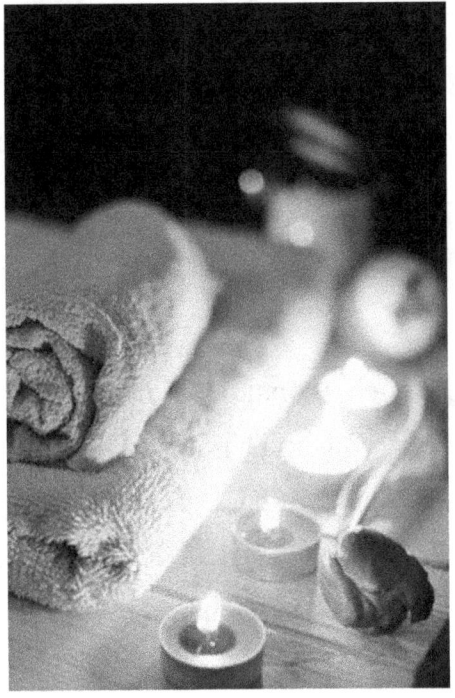

Do you have a stash of scented candles just lying around? Put them to good use. If you're worried about fire-hazards, opt for natural calming scents. This can be supplemented by putting plants and flowers in your room, instead. Just make sure that the size of the plant isn't too big since you don't want it to pose as a distraction.

Tools and Necessities

Aside from comfortable furniture, you will need to make sure your space has all the necessary equipment and tools needed to get started. This may include but isn't limited to:

- Oils, lotions etc.
- Wipes
- Towels
- Massaging tool (we will discuss this in detail in the following chapters)
- Pillows, mats, rugs etc.

Music

For an added touch, consider putting on some relaxing music. Remember, you don't need large sound systems and speakers. A little soft music playing melodiously in the background should do the trick. Soothing jazz music is a popular choice and can add to the relaxing vibes.

Self-Massage: Do's and Don'ts

Before you get started, you ought to brush yourself up on the do's and don'ts of self-massage. Laying down a few ground rules will eliminate the risk of accidents and health concerns.

Do:

- **Make it a part of your routine:** Dedicate out a couple minutes of your day for some pampering. Practice self-massage each day for a week and soon enough you will start to experience the many benefits of self-massaging.
- **Use a clean setting:** This is highly important. Make sure you're using clean towels and tools. Not only will this curb sanitary issues but a cleaner environment will allow you to sit back and relax on a deeper level.
- **Take your time:** Your body is a temple that needs to be explored. Take your time and let your hands intuitively take care of the rest. Apply pressure when necessary or slow down with more soothing strokes – it all comes down to what works best for you.
- **Consider warming oil:** If you have some spare time, consider warming a bottle of oil in a hot water bath. Remember not to apply direct heat as it may result in a fire hazard. Warming up oil is an effective way to enhance your experience.

Don't:

- **Use rancid oil:** If it smells rancid: get rid of it. Invest in high-grade essential oils, cold-pressed oils and aromas for their healing qualities. Remember, you wouldn't eat something that's rotten and molding. So why feed your skin (your body's largest organ) something that's much below par?

- **Clog your drains:** Oil in your shower drain can result in the pipes being clogged. Massage yourself after showering to avoid such problems. If you would rather take a hot bath following your pampering session, flush the drains with warm vinegar at first, to prevent clogs.

- **Expect instant results:** More often than not, people want instant results and are ready to give up the second something does not work out. Understand that self-massage offers both physical and emotional benefits that *take time* to surface. Don't rush — allow your body some time to relax and you will be surprised at the results that can eventually be achieved.

History of Massage

Since this book is about the core essence of massage, it makes sense to back to basics and unveil its history.

As you might well imagine, massage therapy has been around for decades – going back for thousands of years. However, as far as its origins are concerned, the first records of massage can be traced back to China and Egypt.

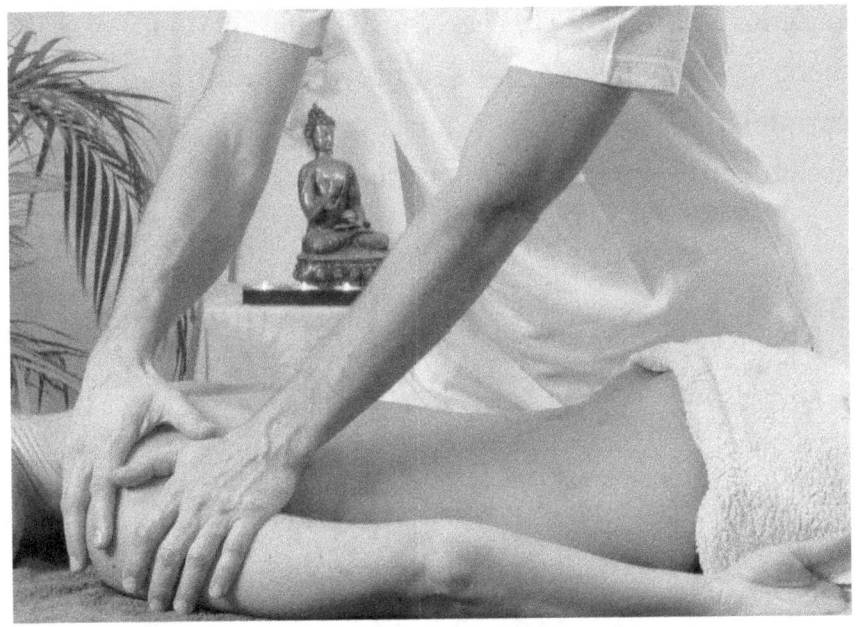

2700 B.C.E: Ancient China

The earliest origin of massage therapy can be dated back to 2700.B.C.E. This can be found preserved in an old Chinese book called "The Yellow Emperor's Classic Book of Internal Medicine." While the book was published in English many

many years later (during the 1900s), it is still now a popular beginner's guide for any student studying acupuncture at school.

2500 B.C.E: Ancient Egypt
In the following 200 years, significant progress was made in the world of massage therapy as the reflexology technique of ancient Egypt had also now been developed. Other than Egypt, this reflexology technique had also been used in ancient Rome and Greece. During that period, massage therapy was popularly used to promote health and combat harmful diseases.This is primarily why reflexology is still used today to treat professional athletes.

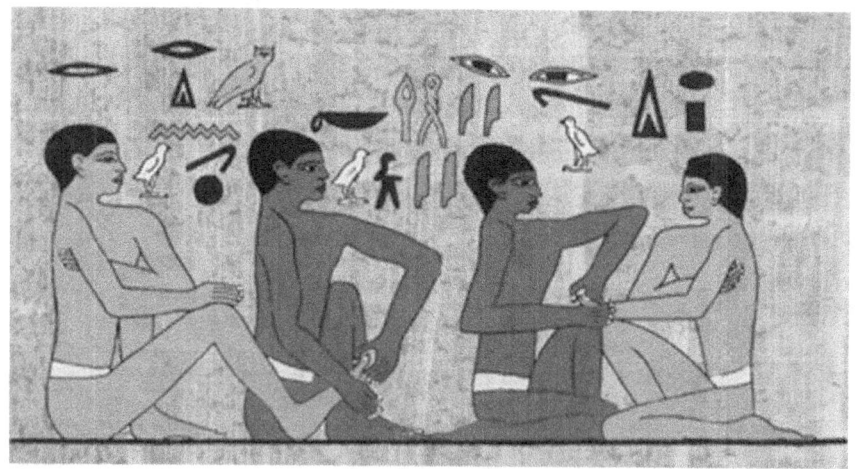

1500 B.C.E: Ayurvedic Medicine
A couple of thousand years later, massage therapy had now grown in popularity in India, along with Ayurvedic medicine. Ayurvedic medicine emphasises on how the soul, body and

mind must all be interconnected in order to function correctly. This symbolic connection paved the way for health experts to be able to explain exactly how Ayurvedic medicine should be practiced.

800-700 B.C.E: Ancient Greece

There's no denying that Greece has one of the most impressive historical cultures in the world. From the Greek Gods, to their obsession with fitness, Greeks pay close attention to physical appearance and how to maintain it.

Massage therapy has remained a common practice in Greece, with experts paying particular attention to getting rid of or reducing knots in muscle tissues.

500 B.C.E: Hippocrates

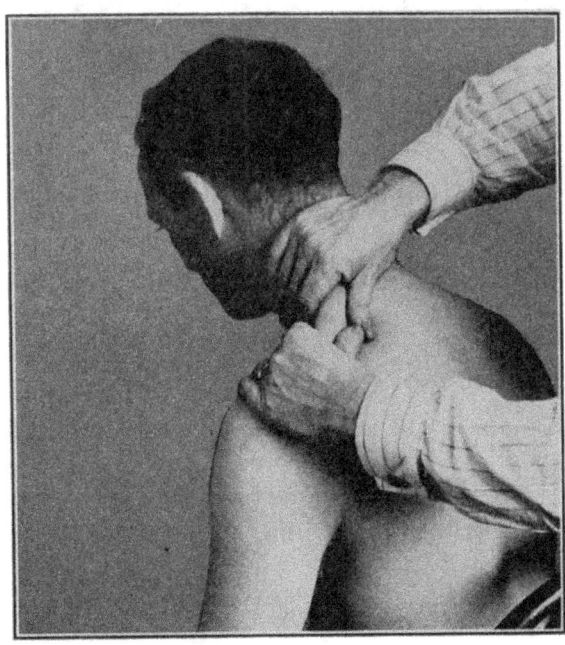

Known as the era of Hippocrates, 500 B.C.E was an important time for modern medicine. As one of the biggest pioneers in regards to modern medicine, Hippocrates' teachings about physical fitness later became practiced worldwide.

Athletes in Greece emphasized the importance of massage for physical health prior to competitions.

Hippocrates was well-known for prescribing it to treat physical ailments. He noticed how applying pressure and rubbing the body in a certain way could speed up healing. He also promoted the idea that a combination of adequate sleep, proper nutrition, exercise and massage would help restore the body to optimal health.

Physicians would encourage the use of special oils and herbs to optimize athletes' performance and to treat a number of medical conditions. Simultaneously, Greek women would use these oils for skin treatments, to enhance their beauty.

1800s: West

The 1800s were a time of considerable progress in the world of massage therapy. During this period a Swedish doctor and gymnast named Per Henril Ling formulated a special technique known as the "Swedish Movement System."

This practice later set a base for Swedish massage, which is still prevalent in the West today. Ling's work was later developed by Johan Georg Mezger, who incorporated hand strokes into the practice.

Swedish massage is one of the most popular treatments in the Western Hemisphere today.

20th Century

Throughout the 20th century, experts have experimented with a number of new methods and techniques in order to more successfully treat physical ailments and concerns. This is highly evident during the aftermath of World War I when patients were treated using specialist massage techniques to prevent shell shock and nerve injury.

However, it should be noted that massage therapy was considered as a sign of luxury, something that was only reserved for the powerful and influential, during the early years of the 20th Century.

During the second half of the 20th century, there were many developments in the world of massage therapy as people increasingly started to opt for natural healing methods to treat their ailments. At this time, industry standards and licensing started to emerge. And thanks to these new rules and regulations, massage therapy was finally recognized as a respectable alternative (not replacement) to medicinal treatment.

Present Day

These days massage therapists emphasize the importance of learning new techniques, whilst also studying and practicing the ancient methods. These ancient traditions serve as building blocks that massage experts can use to help others live a more comfortable life.

Self-Massage Using Aroma Oils

Aromatherapy is another therapeutic practice that is used for holistic healing. It involves the use of selected plant extracts. They are used to make essential oils, which are also known as aroma oils. Each essential oil offers a host of emotional, health and physical benefits. This is primarily why aromatherapy massage has become such a popular phenomenon today.

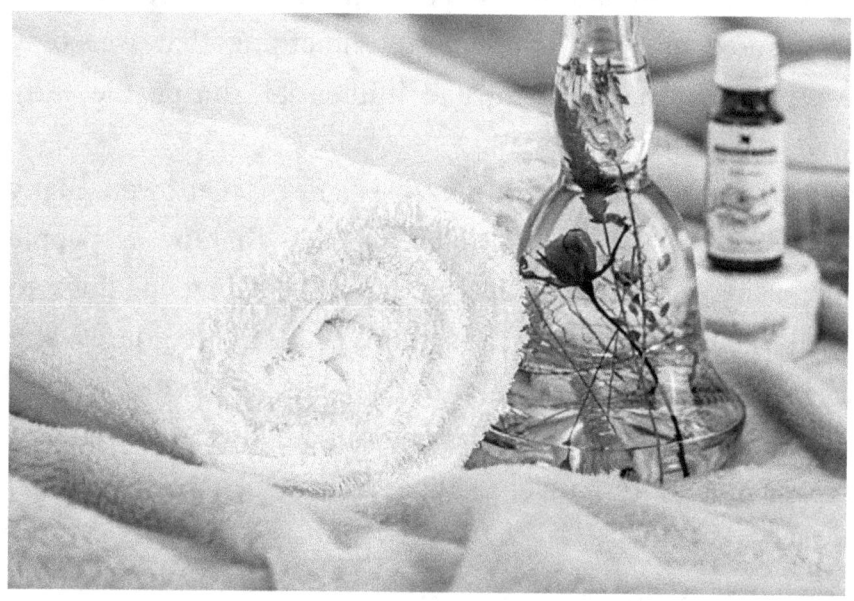

What is Aromatherapy Massage?

This is a type of Swedish massage therapy that incorporates the use of massage oils and lotions that contain essential oils. It should be noted that all essential oils are derived from a plant.

Throughout this treatment, essential oils are being absorbed into the body or inhaled during the massage. These oils are thought to provide healing benefits to the body and mind by targeting the limbic system (a special region in the brain that affects the nervous system).

Benefits of an Aromatherapy Massage

There are many benefits of an aromatherapy massage – most of these benefits are highly similar to that of a Swedish massage — which people often use when treating physical ailments.

A couple of sessions of aromatherapy massage can successfully help treat the following conditions:

- Depression
- Insomnia
- Painful menstrual cramps
- Anxiety
- Symptoms of dementia
- Supportive care for patients suffering from diseases such as cancer

It should be noted that the effectiveness of the massage primarily depends on the type and amount of essential oils used.

Best Essential Oils for Self Massage

Here are some essential oils that are popularly used of massage therapy:

Lavender Oil

Lavender oil is usually a firm favorite when it comes to choosing a calming scent for your aromatherapy massage. It is a balancing oil and is very adaptive in nature. By incorporating a couple of drops of lavender oil to your blend, you can soothe tired muscles and ease backaches and other pains. Simply massage a couple of drops on the affected area and feel your magic hands do wonders. A few massage sessions should do the trick.

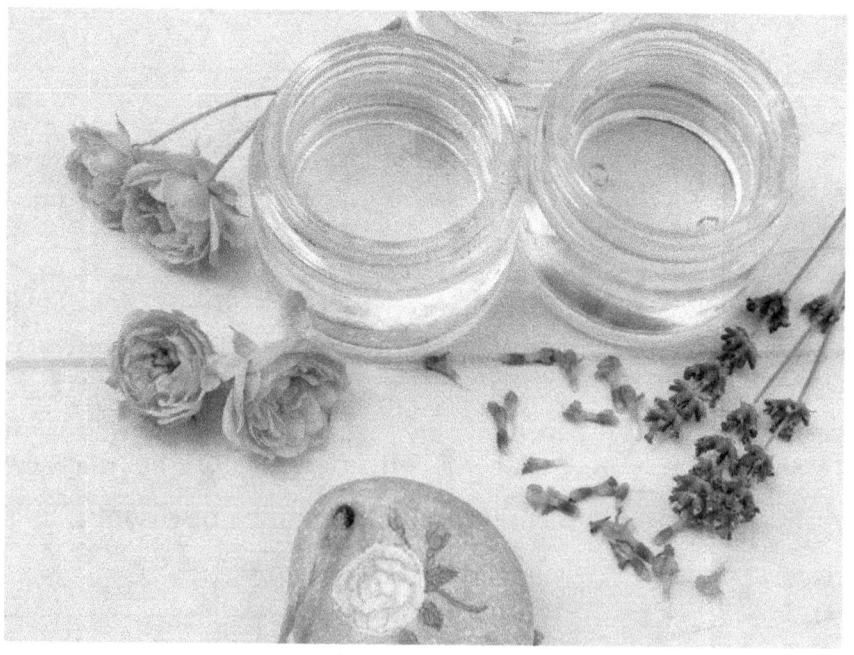

For added benefits, you can also pour a couple of drops of lavender oil into a diffuser. This can help with respiratory problems such as asthma, flu, throat infections, congestion and so on. Massaging lavender oil across your back, chest and neck can also relieve symptoms of respiratory problems.

Above all, lavender oil is an excellent choice for people who have trouble sleeping. Using lavender oil has been estimated to improve sleep up to almost 60%. This is good news for people who suffer with insomnia.

Peppermint Oil

Peppermint oil is another favorite, although it should be used sparingly because of its intense nature.

Because of its cooling properties, adding a few drops of peppermint oil to your blend is great for massaging tired feet. It can also provide relief after a hot day, especially aiding those who are prone to hot flashes.

However, the oil isn't as gentle as one might think, so only use 1-2 drops in a carrier oil and make sure to keep it away from children.

Frankincense Oil

Frankincense is an important essential oil for many reasons: adding 1-2 drops of this oil in your carrier oil blend can be highly effective for soothing coughs and breathing problems.

Frankincense oil also offers a number of anti-inflammatory and anti-depressant properties that can help with a number of ailments.

To double its benefits we suggest blending frankincense oil with lavender oil to alleviate anxiety and curb insomnia. All in all, frankincense oil works as a great carrier oil, which means it can be combined with other essential oils for added benefits.

Precautions for Using Essential Oils

Please understand that essential oils or aromatherapy oils must be used with plenty of care and precaution. Not doing so can lead to adverse reactions that might burn the skin. To eliminate the risk of such instances, here are some basic precautions you should follow:

Diluting the Oil

A general rule of thumb is to restrict the concentration level of the oil to below 5%. Experts recommend that you dilute essential oils before use.

Safe concentration levels may vary among people depending on health condition and age. You must take special measures if you are suffering from an illness or expecting a baby.

The easiest way to dilute an essential oil is to blend it with a carrier oil. Two of the most commonly used oils are coconut or almond. You can decide between the two, depending upon their intended purpose. The safest way to apply essential oils to your skin is to use a vegetable-based carrier oil.

Perform a Patch Test

It is extremely important to perform a patch test before use, to make sure the essential oil does not burn your skin. Start by washing your forearm using an unscented soap. Once the area has dried, rub just a few drops of essential oil on that area. Keep an eye out for any blisters or redness that may be caused by an adverse reaction to the oil. If you do see a reaction, wash the area immediately with warm water and soap. If there are no adverse reactions, you are free to safely use the oil.

Using Essential Oils during Pregnancy

To be absolutely on the safe side, we suggest avoiding all use of essential oils during pregnancy, especially during the first trimester.

Most experts believe that topical essential oils can diffuse into the fetus, causing harm. To avoid any kind of potential danger, regardless of how minor it might be, we suggest avoiding the use of essential oils during pregnancy. Furthermore, we suggest seeking medical advice from a qualified healthcare professional before even considering a use of essential oils during pregnancy.

While topical use of essential oils should be avoided, it may be possible to diffuse certain oils that are deemed as safe (using a diffuser). Some oils that are safe to use: lemon, grapefruit, lavender, and frankincense oil. Women who are breastfeeding should also avoid using essential oils topically as it may cause nausea.

Store Away from Children

Another important precaution is to store these oils out of the reach of children and infants. Keeping in mind that children have thinner skin, they are more susceptible to the potential dangers of essential oils. In the case of oil being ingested by a child, we suggest you call emergency services immediately, or get in touch with the poison center.

Self-Massage Using Essential Oils

There are a number of self-massages that you can perform using essential oils. So what are you waiting for? It's time to light some candles, put on some calming music and create an atmosphere of ambience.

Hand Massage

A relaxing hand massage is just what you need to soothe your tired hands after a long day of typing or handiwork. Start by pouring a liberal amount of essential oils onto your wrists and hands. Use your thumb to gently massage the wrist, knuckles, hands and each finger using gentle, slow circular motions. Apply pressure to the areas that are most sore.

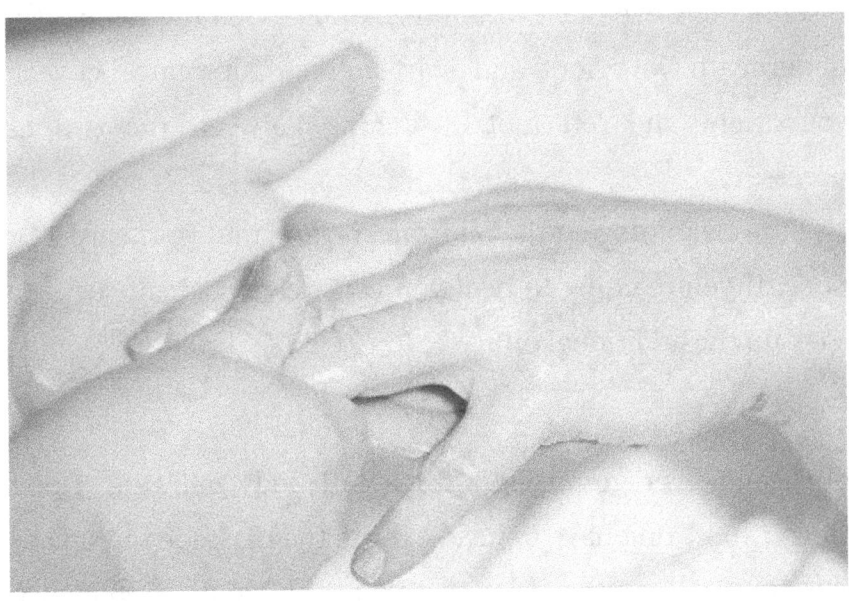

Alternate your movements between clockwise and anti-clockwise motions. Continue massaging your hands and wrists until the oil has penetrated into your skin and feels saturated.

Perform this hand massage in the morning before you head out to work or at the end of a long hard day. Be sure to dry your hands completely once you're done.

Feet Massage

Walking around and standing all day can take its toll on your feet. If this sounds like you, this relaxing foot massage is just what you needed to soothe your tired feet. Start by rinsing your feet in some warm water and then place a towel underneath them. Pour a few of drops of your favorite essential oils over a clean tennis ball. Position the tennis ball underneath your foot and start rolling. Alternate between your right and left foot, switching between the two as necessary.

Use towels to prevent the oil from soaking into your carpet or floor. If you're going to bed, you can wear a pair of socks to soak up the additional oil.

Full Body Massage

You can't ever go wrong with a full body massage. Don't worry; you won't have to head over to the massage therapist's this time. All you need is a set of magic hands — your own should do just fine! Start by generously applying massage oil all over your body.

Sit back and massage the oil gently for about 20 minutes. Start from the tips of your fingers and then move your way up your arms to middle of the body. To really relax your limbs and joints, use long strokes and circular strokes, allowing your skin and muscles to soak up the oil. Once you've reached your abdomen, massage both sides of the body. You can also use some leftover oil to massage your scalp. This is good for your hair. Allow the essential oils to soak in for a couple of minutes.

Consider taking a warm bath to allow the essential oils to work themselves into your muscles. A warm shower can also help soothe those tired muscles, but be sure not to use soap as it will wipe away the essential oils.

Contraindications for Massage

All forms of treatment can cause any number of side effects. While there is not much to worry about as far as massage therapy is concerned, you will have to take special caution if you suffer from a medical condition. If you don't take these factors into account, you may suffer from potentially dangerous injuries.

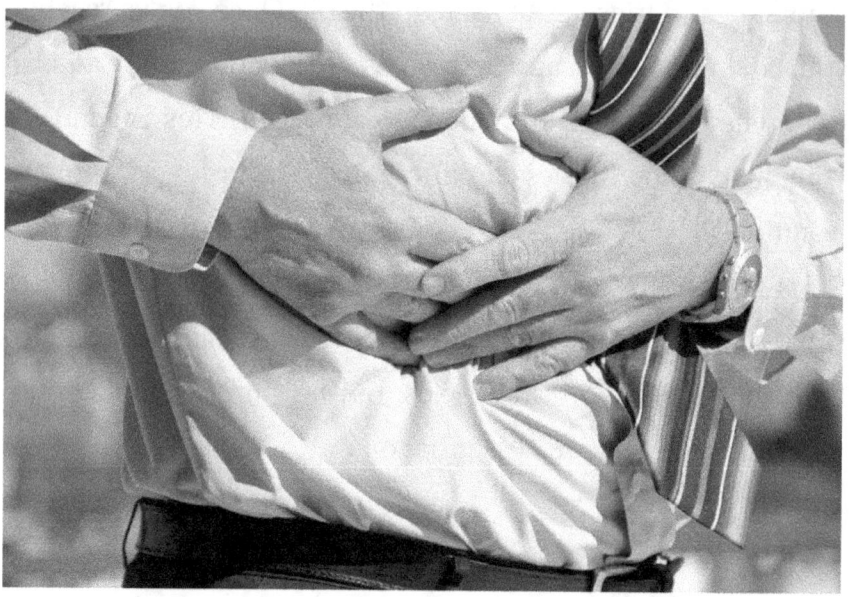

For this reason, we must also be aware of the possible contraindications for a massage.

What are contraindications for a massage?

Contraindications for a massage include any reason that might mean you should avoid getting a massage. These contraindications consist of health problems that could possibly interact negatively with the massage, resulting in severe pain.

You should particularly be aware of absolute contraindications, including:

- Fever
- Diarrhea
- Severe pain
- Kidney disease
- Joint pain etc.

The above mentioned are all conditions in which a massage should absolutely not be performed. However, it should be noted that the intensity or severity of the contraindication can vary, as there are many different categories. Some of the more common categories include:

General Contraindications

In the case of the following contraindications, self-massage or massage therapy must be avoided for a particular time period.

This could include conditions that may require immediate medical attention, an infectious or contagious disease, fever or unstable hypertension.

Local Contraindications

These contraindications only affect certain areas which need to be avoided during a massage. This includes inflammation or swelling of certain parts of the body, aneurysms, recent surgery, any kind of wound, open sores, irritable skin (which may have been caused by an allergic reaction) and other temporary conditions.

Areas to Avoid

It goes without saying that you're not an expert when it comes to giving yourself a massage, and so you ought to stay clear of certain areas of the body. This includes any kind of injury that you may have sustained in the past. As a rule of thumb, it is also recommended that you avoid massaging any area that feels painful.

Here are some of the main areas you should avoid:

Muscle Ruptures

Muscle ruptures are an absolute no-go. These are tears in the muscle that usually occur as a result of extreme stress or due to sudden movements. If you have experienced a muscle rupture while working out or because of any other kind of injury, we suggest you visit the doctor immediately. This is because all muscle ruptures are expected to bleed within 48 to 72, once the injury has taken place.

Because of this, do not massage the affected area as it is likely to become inflamed and sensitive.

Burns

Did you spend a lovely weekend at the beach but ended up with a bad sunburn? Apply some aloe vera gel and leave the affected area alone. The same goes for if you have experienced a kitchen burn caused by fire, hot water or friction. Be sure not to massage that particular area or perhaps put some cold on it (e.g. apply wet cold towel or use running cold water) for some relief. Burns require adequate time for healing and should not be massaged, especially if you are still experiencing pain.

Tendon Ruptures

Depending on the severity of the injury, tendon ruptures can be incredibly painful. As a result, you should avoid massaging the affected area at all costs. If the pain is unbearable, you may have to opt for surgery. We advise you seek medical help and avoid touching the sensitive areas of your tendons which of course, means also abstaining from massages for some time.

Bumps

Have you noticed a strange bump on your shoulder or any other part of the body? Unless you have gotten it checked by the doctor, it's best you leave it alone. Often these bumps are a result of fatty tissues and muscle spasms. Avoid massaging the area around the bump and seek appropriate medical assessment to put your mind at rest and to rule out the chances of it being a harmful disease.

Hand Self-Massaging Techniques

There are a number of self-massaging techniques that you can practice simply using your own hands! While there are many different massage tools (we will discuss these in the upcoming chapters), using your hands in the most natural and authentic way to ease tensions and relax your muscles can be just as effective. Unlike using tennis balls and other tools, your hands will offer your muscles just the right amount of precision and pressure necessary.

The only downside is that your hands may tire after a couple of minutes. Rest assured, you can always keep your massage sessions short to address this problem and avoid discomfort.

Some areas that are ideal for your hands include your arms, shoulders and neck. Here are some techniques that you can use for self-massaging:

Finger Technique

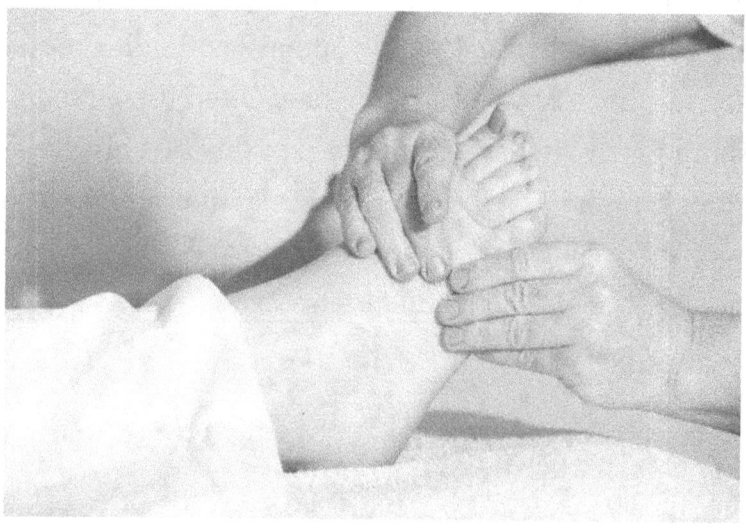

Position your fingertips on the area that you wish to massage; the trick is to locate sore or tender spots.

Gently apply pressure on the affected spot and slowly move your fingers around the particular area. Make sure your fingers are making contact with the muscle affected.

The best part about using your fingers is that it offers a precise range of motion and accurately hits the spot.

Once you have finished working on the tenderest part, the next step is to release tension and go back to where you began the massage. Keeping your strokes to a maximum of fifteen is a good call, but if you find you prefer just five strokes, then this pattern should work fine too.

A good trick is to use your other hand to support your massaging hand whenever possible. Simultaneously this will protect your joints and will allow you to exert more pressure when needed.

Knuckle Technique

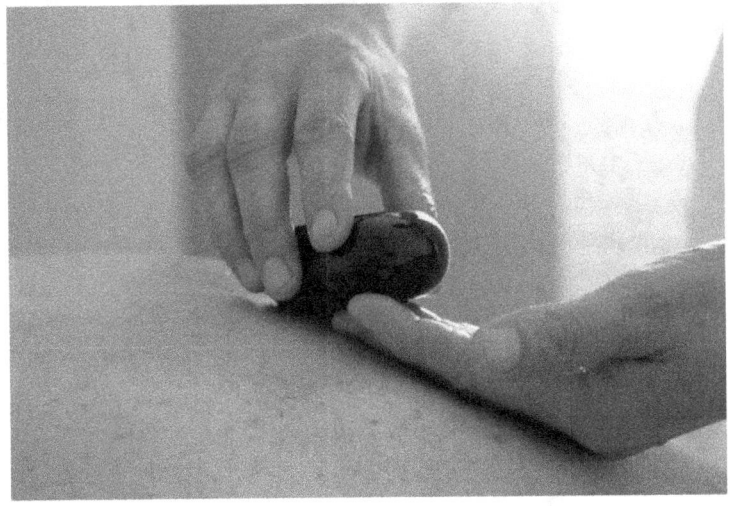

Aside from your fingers, using your knuckles is the next best way to apply pressure and massage various parts of your body. To use this technique, make a fist (without closing your fingers too tightly), slide your knuckles over the affected area and vary the pressure according to your personal preference. We advise you use slow strokes, especially when dealing with tender areas.

We recommend using this technique while massaging your hands and forearms.

Thumb Index Finger Technique

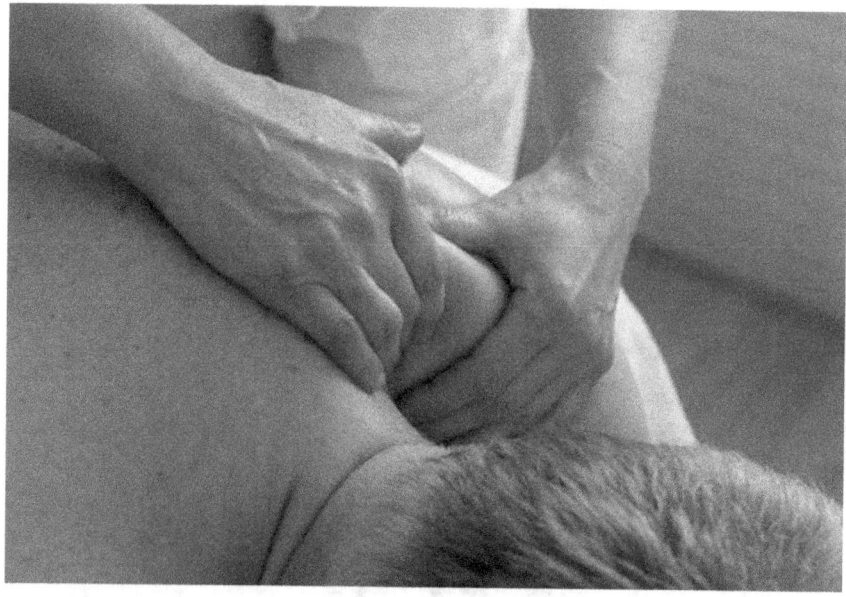

As the name indicates, this technique involves rolling the affected area between your thumb and index finger. This technique is great for targeting small muscle groups.

However, it should only be reserved for muscles that can be pulled and pinched easily.

Roll and gently pinch the desired area about 5 to 10 times between your fingers. On the downside, this self-massage technique can tire your hands rather quickly, so keep your sessions short whenever necessary.

Thumb Technique

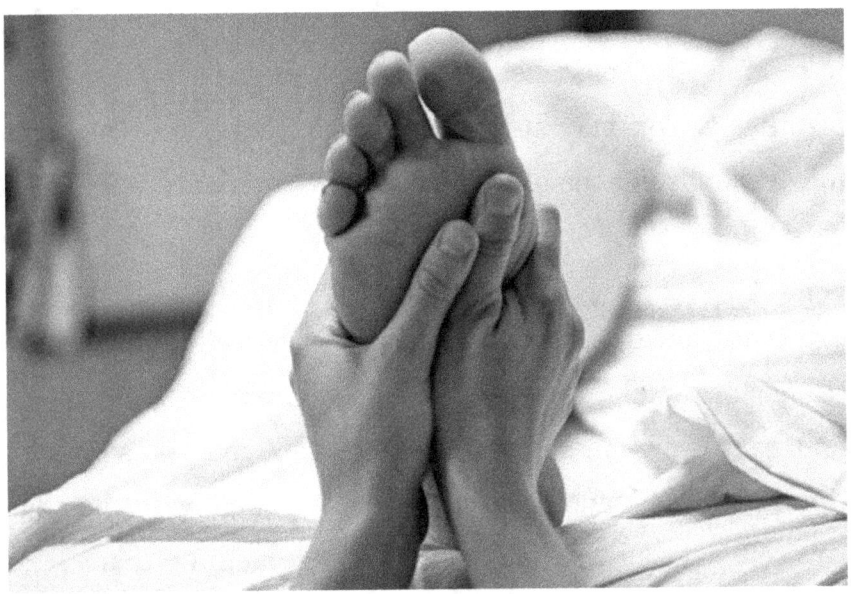

The thumb technique is quite similar to the finger technique and is great for massaging small, targeted areas. This technique involves applying pressure to the affected area but make sure to be gentle and only use about 10 to 15 strokes per muscle group. Be sure to support your thumb using your index finger. This will keep your joint stable and will prevent your thumb from getting tired out.

How to Prepare Yourself for a Massage

Before we list some of our amazing self-massage techniques, you will first have to prepare yourself first. This is crucial if you want to enjoy a relaxing massage therapy session without any disturbances or worries.

Pay attention to the following guidelines to benefit as much as possible from your relaxing session. It is also a good idea to reserve your massage therapy sessions for around the end of the day. You may also schedule your pampering sessions for weekends, for the ultimate massage experience.

Eat Lightly

Trust us, you don't want to massage yourself on a bloated stomach, so make sure you have had your meal about 2 to 3 hours prior the massage session. This will give you sufficient time to unwind and relax. If you are planning to massage yourself right after lunch, you can eat something that's light and does not have too many calories. It is also recommended you drink plenty of water – but not too much — to avoid bloating.

Stay Hydrated

We cannot emphasize enough how crucial it is to drink plenty of water. Drinking water is important for eliminating toxins from the body during massage therapy, ensuring it is released through the body's circulation. If drinking a lot of water is too boring for you, you can also opt for herbal tea or green tea. On the other hand, try to avoid drinking sugary or caffeinated drinks such as teas and coffees.

Switch off Your Phone

Before beginning the massage, switch off your phone or at least put it in silent mode. Seeing a work email suddenly pop up on your screen may suddenly cause you to spring up in a state of panic. This would defeat the whole purpose of giving yourself a massage, which is to relax and relieve stress.

To make this massage session more enjoyable, switch off your phone and try to relax and unwind. We also recommend giving yourself a break from social media, while you're at it.

Dress Comfortably

Because a massage only requires contact with skin, many undermine the importance of wearing comfortable clothes. Here's the thing; wearing comfortable clothes will allow better movement and allow you to enjoy the sensations of massage therapy in a more relaxed state than if you were wearing tight or uncomfortable clothes. This is most important when it comes to footwear. We suggest staying clear of high heels following your massage.

Plan Your Session

Plan a day of pampering so that you have something to look forward to. Clear your schedule and get those massage oils ready. Having to run out for an urgent task might spring your mind into panic and kill those peaceful vibes altogether. Before you lie down to pamper yourself, try to take deep breaths and allow your mind to relax. Make sure the room you have chosen is peaceful and quiet.

After the Massage

It is worth noting that massage oils might have a detoxing effect on your body, resulting in dehydration. To avoid this, we suggest drinking plenty of water.

If you have chosen a massage therapy that uses oils, allow the oils to sink into your body, unless you have other plans that day. If you do have to leave, you will need to take a shower and wash away any oil left on your skin. If this seems like too much of a hassle, you can buy some dry oil instead, which does not leave any residue behind.

Your feet might begin to feel a little sore after the massage. Understand that this is nothing to be worried about, since it is caused by the influx of lactic acid in the body. This can easily be cured by lying down for a while or by drinking a lot of water, which will flush the lactic acid out of the body.

Self-Massage Techniques to Relieve Stress

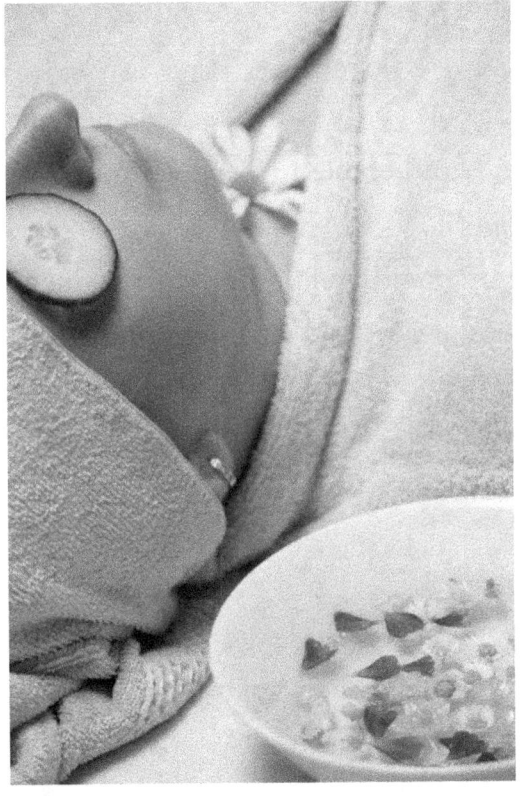

Whether you come home after a long day at work or have finally been able to put your little one to sleep, self-massage is an essential stress releasing activity that everybody should practice. However, not everybody has the time nor the finances to visit a professional massage therapist, which is why learning self-massage techniques can be a life-saver.

Here are a few simple self-massage techniques that you can practice at home:

Lower Back

Massaging the lower back can be a challenging experience, since you may not be able to reach certain areas. The lower back is susceptible to all kinds of muscle knots, often caused by poor posture or sitting at a desk for too long. Fortunately, there are a number of massage tools that can help get ease muscle knots and back pain. One of these tools is an S-shaped trigger point massager.

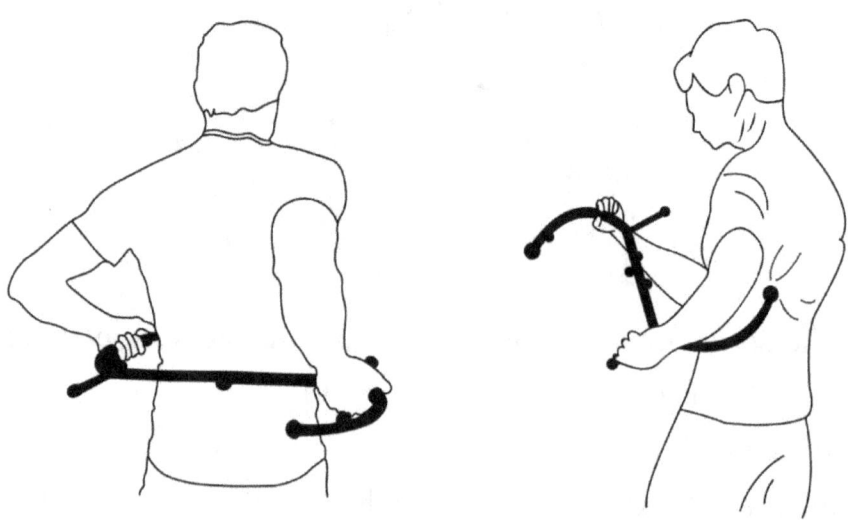

The lower back withstands an immense amount of stress and pressure, especially if you're not in the habit of maintaining a good posture. To massage your back, you will need an S-shaped trigger point massage tool. Hook this tool over your shoulder to reach your back muscles. Make sure you hold the handles in a comfortable position, and ensure that it can get to the desired muscle areas.

As you use the massage tool, push it towards the affected spot, and then pull it away. Repeat this on the opposite side of your body. Then position the end of the massager below the arch of your left arm. Apply pressure wherever you feel necessary.

Keep in mind that you shouldn't directly apply pressure to your spine. If you wish to target a specific area in the lower back, simply prolong the pressure applied to this particular area, instead of intensifying pressure. This technique will reduce the chances of pain.

To make your massage even more stress relieving, take slow deep breathes with each stroke. If needed, you can also use this tool to apply pressure to the hips, chest, feet and arm areas.

Feet

Walking around all day on uncomfortable shoes can add a lot of strain to our feet. They often undergo a considerable amount of stress that can also take a toll on our well-being. Aside from giving them a nice warm foot bath, you can relax your feet with a soothing massage.

Refloxology is linked to healing your entire body through the soles of your feet. The sole has about 200,000 nerve endings, making it incredibly sensitive. The sole is also believed to have several reflex points, which are known to stimulate other organs and address various different health conditions.

Use a Foot Massager

For added convenience, consider using a foot massager. While this is a slightly more costly option, investing in a foot massager can be worth it in the long run, especially if you have stiff feet or suffer from arthritis.

You can either invest in an electronic or manual model. A manual model typically features pointed knobs or wooden rollers that are designed to stimulate foot muscles. On the other hand, an electronic device will include much more advanced features such as heat technology for better results.

Self-Massage Using a Tennis Ball

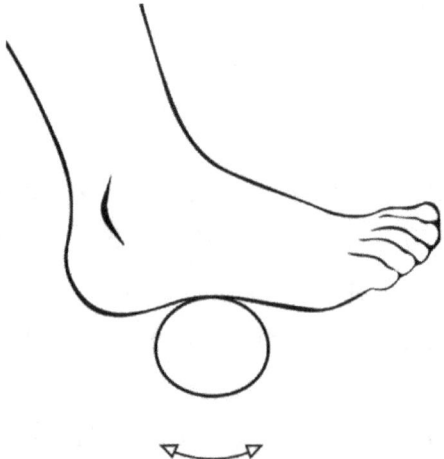

Tennis balls are among the most popular tools used for self-massaging. This technique is especially beneficial for those who have tired and sore feet. Simply take a clean tennis ball and position it under your foot. Roll the tennis ball back and forth with your feet, applying additional pressure wherever necessary.

What's great about this massage technique is that you can massage your feet discretely while at work, without anyone even noticing!

Calves

Use a foam roller to massage tired legs and calves.

If you walk around in high heels all day, then it's crucial that you find a way to release the tension and tightness in your hamstrings and calves that will have built up during the day. Sports massage experts often emphasize on the importance of massaging overlooked muscle groups, such as the calves, while training. Continual neglect of your calves and ankle joints can cause problems in the future.

Begin by placing a long foam roller (ideally the length of your calf muscles) underneath your calves.

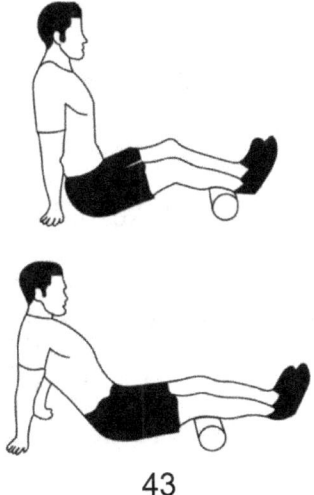

Position the foam roller and support yourself using your palms. Next, roll the foam roller underneath your legs and calves. Slowly move your legs up and down as much as you like. Practice this movement to release tension and improve flexibility of calf muscles.

Hands & Wrists

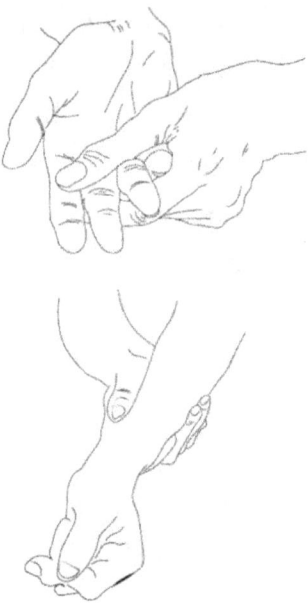

In everyday life our hands take quite a beating. Whether we're cooking, typing, or driving; our hands are constantly in motion. Massaging your hands during times of stress can help release tension and promote feelings of relaxation. Fortunately, performing a hand massage is not too difficult and can also be practiced in an office environment, whenever you are feeling stressed out.

For instant stress relief, massage the fleshy spot that lies between your index finger and your thumb. This is known to be a key acupressure point that releases a feeling of relaxation when massaged. Use your thumb to slowly massage the spot for a couple of seconds, using slow circular motions.

Move your focus to the base of your hand and massage the area above the wrist, applying a slight pressure to relieve tension.

Massaging the Wrists

Similar to hands, wrists also take quite a beating, as a consequence of all the typing we do, at the office and at home. The good news is that a tennis or massage ball can prove quite handy when it comes to massaging your wrist.

While there are numerous ways to massage your wrist, using a tennis ball is one of the most effective ways to gain relief from stress. Simply place a tennis ball on a clean, hard surface. Position your wrist on top of the tennis ball, making sure it is placed underneath your palm. Now spread your fingers and gently roll the ball towards the bottom of your forearm (and back again).

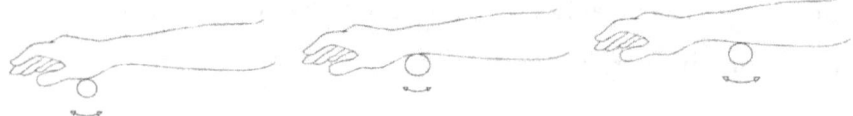

Make sure to have a good handle on the amount of pressure you apply, as putting too much pressure on the joints may result in numbness. Use this technique to massage your wrists for about 15 minutes.

Neck And Shoulders

Massaging your neck and shoulders is the easiest way to relieve stress when you are not feeling well or are experiencing pain.

More often than not, stress can find its way into your neck and shoulder muscles.

To massage your shoulders, begin by gently massaging your right shoulder using slow circular motions, rubbing your tired muscles using your index or middle fingers. Place the opposite hand on top of your head to ensure stability and that your hand doesn't wobble. Alternate with your left shoulder when you're done massaging your right.

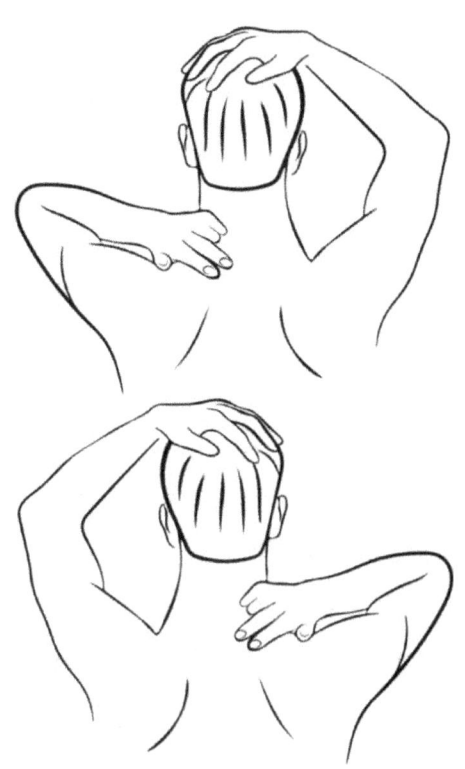

Face & Head

Working too late or high stress levels can result in painful headaches. Relaxing head massages are some of the best ways to relieve muscle tension. Start by gently massaging your temples with your fingers using circular motions. Be sure not to rub the skin with your fingers, but rather gently move the scalp back and forth, and then stroke your fingers around the head band.

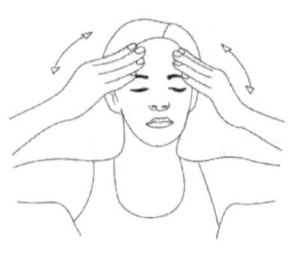 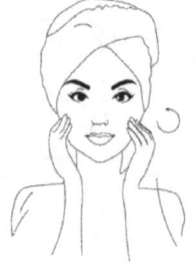 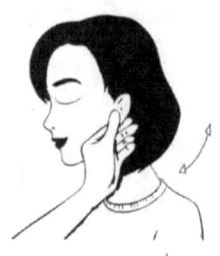

Using both hands, cater to each side of your head. When your fingers meet at the top of the scalp, stop and reverse the direction. Inhaling deeply and relaxing your entire body should also help with this process.

Tired eyes and cheekbones could often do with some pampering. Fortunately there are several different ways you can relieve tension in these areas. Begin by resting the heels of your palms on the side of your face, positioning your hands just above your cheeks. Very gently, pull down the skin covering your forehead and skull, with your fingertips, while slowly pushing up the area under your palms.

Gently repeat this movement, alternately releasing and contacting your palms and fingers. Gently pulling your ears is another great way to release tension.

Tools for Self-Massage

When it comes to a soothing session of self-massage, most people assume that they can only use their hands, but this is a myth. There are a number of tools that you can invest in to give yourself a pampering massage.

Using the right self-massage tools will allow you to apply moderate amounts of pressure on affected areas for longer periods of time. Massaging for a long amount of time might not be possible when using your hands alone, as they tend to tire more easily. Rest assured, you don't have to invest in a bundle of the most expensive massage tools in the market. In the following list, we have included some of the most useful tools for self-massage:

Massage Ball

Massage balls have been around since ancient times and so this particular tool has certainly evolved over the years. Thousands of years ago, the most ancient cultures would use chilled or warm stones for massage.

Today, massage balls are called by a variety of names – 'yoga balls', 'myofascial release balls' or 'mobility balls'.

Regardless of what you call them, these balls do a fantastic job of isolating the affected area and giving it the care and attention needed for effective treatment. A smooth, round ball can give your body a deep tissue massage through providing just the right amount of pressure needed.

Another benefit of using a massage ball is that you can discreetly place it on your desk without attracting too much attention.

Here are a few types of massage balls you can buy for your practice:

Tennis Ball

An ordinary tennis ball can do wonders for your sore muscles. A few possible uses for a tennis ball during massage have already been listed in this book, and there are many more. These lightweight balls can help apply just the right amount of pressure to your trigger points without resulting in any injuries. On the downside, tennis balls are hallow are may become deformed after a few days of use. This is why we recommend you invest in an entire pack for convenience.

Lacrosse Ball

This is another ball that definitely works well for self-massage. Unlike a tennis ball, a Lacrosse ball is relatively hard and dense – meaning that it won't soften when pressure is applied. This increases its usability in the long run. If used correctly, lacrosse balls can do an excellent job in relieving pain, especially when it comes to healing sore muscles.

This ball is recommended for self-myofascial release. The fascia is a thin layer of connective tissue that covers various organs and muscles in the body. It is also responsible for connecting different muscle groups. In case of any kind of tear, users may experience significant pain and difficulty in moving. Should you experience any sort of pain (more than just the usual ache of tired muscles), do get in touch with a trained medical professional for advice and/or treatment.

Massage Ball with Spikes

These spiky massage are made to focus on different areas of the body by loosening up the muscle tissue. The spikes also improve blood circulation and relax sore muscles. However, not everybody is a fan of their spiky texture as using them can feel uncomfortable at first. Speaking to a professional is recommended before using this particular tool, especially if you are suffering from muscle tear. On the bright side, this massage tool does an excellent job of simultaneously improving blood flow and of stimulating muscle reflexes.

Lightweight vs. Heavy Massage Balls

It is worth mentioning that everybody has their own special needs and requirements when it comes to massage. Some may require more pressure on their muscles, while others may prefer a soft tissue massage without any fancy instruments. Generally, it is beneficial to start your massage routine with a lightweight tennis ball and gradually move to a heavier ball.

People with special physical needs may benefit from a solid ball rather than inflatable one, because of the added weight. It makes the job easier because a solid ball is much easier to maneuver and reacts in a more predictable way when you apply pressure to it.

51

Heating Pad

A heating pad is an important tool that can take your massage therapy to the next level. You can use a heating pad prior your massage to loosen tension and improve blood flow in the particular area.

Massage experts have confirmed that heat therapy can play an active role in providing relaxation and comfort. Aside from relieving pain and muscle soreness, heat pad can also be used to relax muscles after working out or to ease over-exertion. In the long run doing so can prevent muscle spasms and soothe body stiffness. However, purchasing a cold pack for the summer months can also be beneficial when temperatures are high.

How does a heating pad work?

So here's how it works, heat dilates the blood vessels that suffuse the muscles. This in turn promotes and encourages the flow of oxygen, increasing the transportation of nutrients. This helps damaged muscle tissue to heal as sensory receptors are stimulated, which in turn, relieves discomfort.

Additionally, applying heat on the affected area facilitates the movement and stretching of soft tissues. All of which improve flexibility and this is highly important for a healthy body.

Depending on your budget, you can invest in a regular heating pad or opt for something that comes with fancy bells and whistles. We recommend you invest in a pad that has a large surface area – this will make it easier for you to target large areas such as the abdomen, lower back and legs.

Some other inexpensive alternatives to heat therapy include hot baths, heat wraps and warm gel packs.

Trigger Point Back Massager

Massaging your hands and feet might seem relatively easy. But what should you do when you can't reach that aching spot on your back? Rest assured, there are a plethora of tools that will make it easier to reach tough spots.

In this case, a trigger point back massager is just what you need. This tool typically features several nodules that make access to various parts of the body you wouldn't otherwise be able to massage, possible. This tool is a life saver for those who wish to seek relief from stress and dissolve pain in hard to reach places.

We recommend you invest in an S-shaped tool, similar to the example illustrated earlier on, for lower back massage. This simple tool can be used by practically anyone. The therapy knobs situated across the frame are designed to apply pressure on sensory receptors various body parts including the back, hips, shoulders, neck, etc. When these receptors are stimulated, tension is relieved.

Foot Massager

For days when you're too tired to give yourself a massage a foot massager should work wonders with minimal effort. In this case your choice of purchase will undoubtedly depend on your budget. A foot massager will provide you the luxury of enjoying a good massage anytime your feet are aching. This is a great investment for those who are always on their feet and constantly standing because of their job.

Foot massage is mostly linked to reflexology and when the right parts are targeted result in a reduced amount of stress, increased bouts of energy along with improved concentration: It may even cause relief for certain ailments. To reap the most benefits from your new tool, we recommend investing in an electric foot massager.

Foam Roller

If you workout at the gym or take yoga classes, then you're probably familiar with using this kind of apparatus. The humble foam roller makes a great massage tool for myofascial release. This causes contracted muscles to relax, improving blood flow in various areas of the body, resulting in easy movement. This also reduces internal rubbing of body parts and improves the flow of nutrients from the blood into the body.

Self-massage using a foam roller can improve your range of motion and this in turn reduces chances of injury. Additionally, self-massage techniques using a foam roller can also improve healing and decrease recovery time. It can also help warm up your muscles before a workout. And since a foam roller is not too large in size, it can conveniently be carried in your workout bag, or kept in the boot of your car, so it is always there when you need it.

Conclusion

Thank you for reading *Self-Massage: How To Relieve Stress With Self-Massaging Techniques*. We hope this eBook has helped you to overcome stress through using its self-massage techniques. In this highly stressful and stimulating world, it is essential to take your time — to relax and unwind every once in a while. It's perfectly possible, if you are not looking to use a professional massage therapist, to unwind at home.

With this eBook, we hoped to share some simple massage techniques that you can incorporate into your daily life. Most of the self-massage techniques that we have mentioned are incredibly easy to perform. Some of these massages, particularly those meant for the hand and feet areas, can be discreetly performed, even while you're at work. Remember, the best way to combat stress is to create a peaceful environment for yourself.

Make sure you stay safe and seek help from a professional should a health problem get worse at any point in time.

If this eBook has proven to be handy for you, please don't forget to leave a positive review. Thanks again!

www.ingramcontent.com/pod-product-compliance
Lightning Source LLC
Chambersburg PA
CBHW072120280526
45788CB00006B/2567